Dietary Fats

BALANCING
HEALTH & FLAVOR

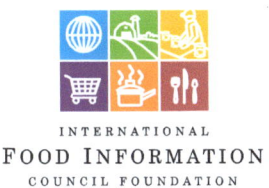

INTERNATIONAL
FOOD INFORMATION
COUNCIL FOUNDATION

Table of Contents

Dietary Fat: The Misunderstood Nutrient

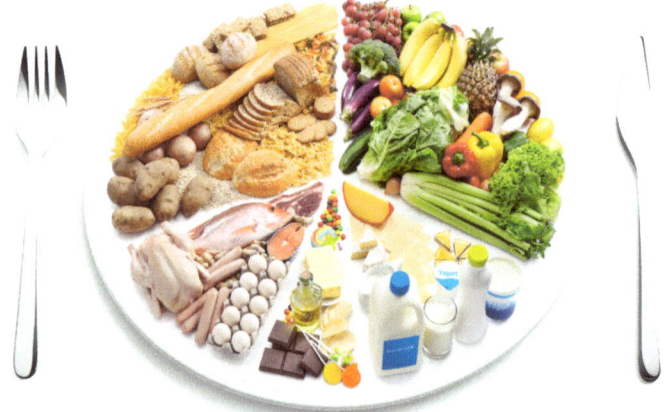

Research on dietary fats and health has advanced considerably in recent years, revealing their complex and critical roles in overall health and well-being.

The misperception that fats are generally unhealthy is slowly being corrected as scientific evidence regarding the healthfulness of unsaturated fatty acids is more widely communicated. As consumer understanding and interest progress, questions are also evolving from "How do I get less?" to "How do I get the best?"

A strong understanding of fats in foods and their component fatty acids is essential for guiding consumers towards a healthful eating

What are dietary fats?

Fats in foods are combinations of many different fatty acids that all play specific roles in the body.

pattern. Mixing the right measure of unsaturated fatty acids and a dash of kitchen wisdom will help consumers to enjoy foods that are both healthful and tasty.

Are all fats the same?

Understanding the basics of fats and fatty acids will help to answer this question. Some of the answers may be surprising! Fats are a group of water insoluble compounds. Fats in foods are made up of a blend of fatty acids, even though foods often become associated with only one type (such as olive oil for monounsaturated fatty acids (MUFA) or butter for saturated fatty acids).

Fatty acid molecules vary in length, shape, and degree of saturation. These differences impart the characteristics of fats, and relate directly to their functions in food and the body.

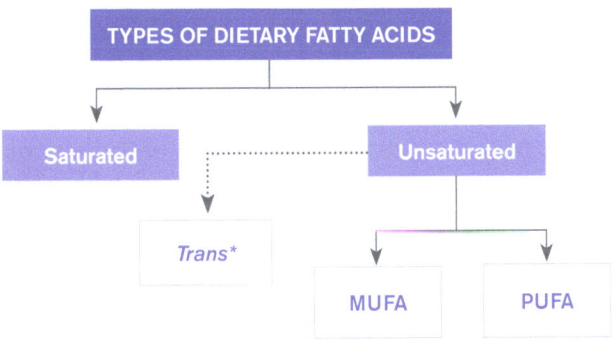

Trans fatty acids are shown in the chart with a dotted line, because although they are technically unsaturated, those that are formed through partial hydrogenation have food and health properties that are more characteristic of saturated fats. See text for further discussion.

Fatty acids can be either saturated or unsaturated. Saturated fatty acids have no double bonds between the carbon atoms, therefore they can be "saturated" with hydrogen atoms (i.e., bond with the maximum number of hydrogen atoms). Unsaturated fatty acids have double bonds within the carbon chain, which causes the structure to bend, similar to how an arm bends at the elbow. This bending limits

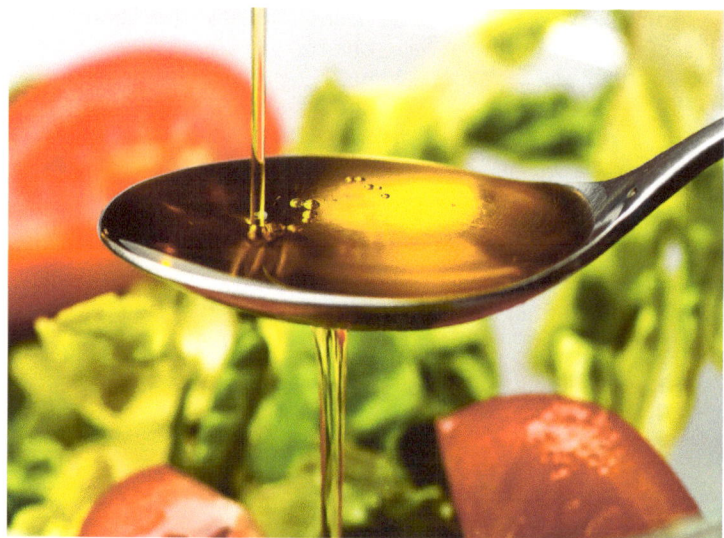

the number of hydrogen atoms that can bind to the carbon atoms, so the molecule is "unsaturated." Unsaturated fatty acids with one double bond are called monounsaturated fatty acids (MUFAs), and those with more than one double bond are called polyunsaturated fatty acids (PUFAs).

PUFAs are further defined as omega-3 and omega-6 fatty acids based on where the first double bond is found within the carbon chain. Two types of PUFA are essential, meaning they must be consumed in the diet because the human body cannot produce them. The essential fatty acids are linoleic acid, which is an omega-6 fatty acid, and alpha-linolenic acid, which is an omega-3 fatty acid.

Often referred to as "solid fats," fats high in saturated fatty acids are typically solid and more stable at room temperature, making them generally less prone to spoilage or oxidation compared to liquid oils; however, there are many notable exceptions. Saturated fatty acids are primarily found in animal products such as meats, dairy, and eggs, but also found in fully hydrogenated vegetable oils and tropical oils, such as palm and coconut.

Unsaturated fatty acids are more liquid than saturated fatty acids at room temperature. Vegetable- or plant-derived oils primarily contain unsaturated fatty acids. The high level of unsaturated fatty acids in liquid oils makes them beneficial for our health, but can also make them more vulnerable to spoilage or oxidation both in foods and in the body.

There are two kinds of *trans* fatty acids. They are found in small amounts in foods from ruminant animals, such as cows and sheep. They are also produced in liquid oils that are partially hydrogenated to improve stability and functionality of the oil when used as a food ingredient. Because they can be solid at room temperature, they are also referred to as "solid fats." Research has shown that *trans* fatty acids, although not fully saturated, can increase risk factors associated with cardiovascular disease. Therefore, agricultural and food science are being used to develop oils and fats that are stable in foods and also beneficial for human health.

In food

Fats, whether saturated or unsaturated, play many roles in foods. Fats affect food appearance (a shiny or glossy look) and texture (crispness, density, flakiness), aid in the browning process, absorb and transport flavors, and transfer heat to food. Liquid oils, with higher levels of unsaturated fatty acids, are well-suited for foods that are liquid, such as salad dressings and sauces. They also work well in sautéing or frying. Solid fats tend to work better in some baking and frying methods with their contribution to texture and stability, although liquid oils are increasingly used in baking with success.

There are many whole foods that are rich sources of healthy unsaturated fatty acids, such as soybeans, olives, avocado, nuts, peanuts, seeds, and certain seafood. From these foods, oils, flours, milks, cheeses, and other foods are produced for use in your home kitchen or as an ingredient in processed foods. While oils that are partially hydrogenated contain *trans* fatty acids, this process is used much less often in processed foods today.

A critical point to understand is that any food with fat contains an array of fatty acids, nearly always a blend of saturated and unsaturated fats, and many other important nutrients. Knowing the primary fatty acid in a food can help when making both culinary and health decisions, but rarely should be the only factor taken into account. See the section on Blending Form and Function in the Kitchen for additional information on cooking with different types of fats.

In the body

Fats have even more diverse functions in the human body. Fat is an integral component of all cell membranes, as well as brain and nervous tissue. About 60% of the brain is made up of fat. In fact, lower levels of brain fat alter brain function and certain fats are critical for proper visual and cognitive development in young infants. Fat is involved in transportation and storage of the fat soluble vitamins A, D, E, and K, and production and proper functioning of key hormones that regulate blood pressure, blood clotting, immune function, and smooth muscle contraction.

Too little dietary fat, especially PUFAs, results in a decrease in fat soluble vitamin availability, may reduce HDL cholesterol (good cholesterol), and interferes with critical body processes. Diets low in omega-3 PUFA may increase the negative cardiovascular impact of high LDL cholesterol (bad cholesterol), contribute to poor blood clotting, and reduce inflammatory responses. Without adequate omega-3

PUFA and vitamin E, cell membranes may become damaged, cell DNA altered, and cellular function disrupted.

Dietary fat has 9 kcal/g, being more calorically dense than both carbohydrates and fat at 4 kcal/g. Thus, managing intake of dietary fat may require closer attention to ensure individual calorie needs are not exceeded. High-fat diets have been correlated with increased risk of heart disease, hypertension, diabetes, and orthopedic problems. However, the importance of dietary fat for health, especially unsaturated fatty acids, is now widely recognized. It's about balance, replacing saturated and *trans* with unsaturated fatty acids, and seeking foods that are also rich in other important nutrients.

How much fat do we need?

While the Food and Nutrition Board of the Institute of Medicine determined in 2002 that healthy Americans should consume approximately 20-35% of calories (44 to 78 g for a 2000-calorie diet) from total fat, the 2010 Dietary Guidelines for Americans noted that most Americans get too much saturated and *trans* fatty acids, and not enough unsaturated fatty acids. Therefore, the focus is on replacing saturated and *trans* fatty acids for unsaturated, not reducing total fat intake.

Dietary Fat Intake Recommendations	2000 kcal/d
Total fat, 20-35% kcal	44-78 g/d
Saturated fatty acids	22 g/d
< 10% kcal With CVD risk, < 7% kcal	15 g/d
Trans fatty acids	As low as possible
Cholesterol	≤ 300 mg/d
Omega 3 fatty acids	0.5-1.0 g/d
SOURCES: Dietary Reference Intakes, Food and Nutrition Board, Institute of Medicine, 2002/5; Dietary Guidelines for Americans, 2010; American Heart Association	

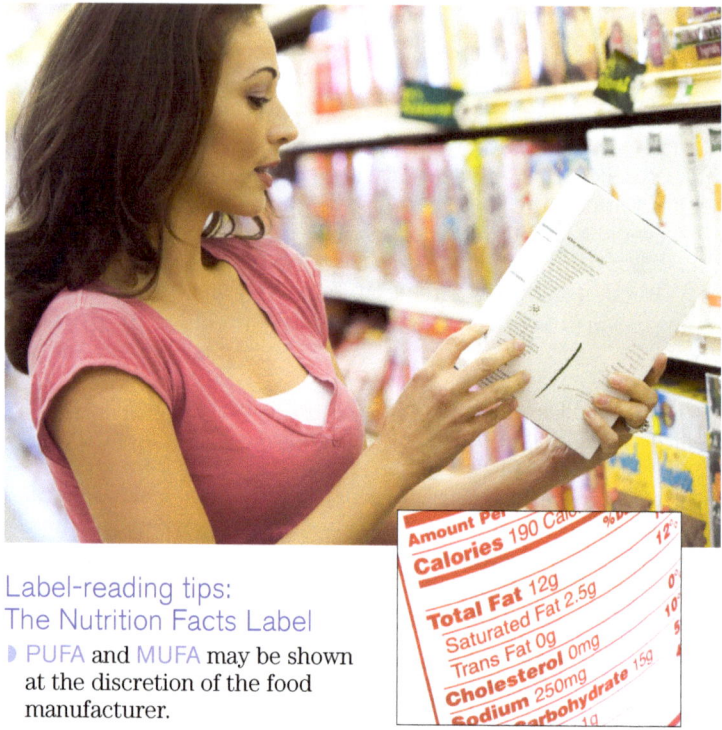

Label-reading tips:
The Nutrition Facts Label

▶ PUFA and MUFA may be shown at the discretion of the food manufacturer.

▶ To determine the amount of unsaturated fat in a food, subtract saturated and *trans* from total fat.

▶ Omega-3 fatty acids are not listed in the Nutrition Facts Label, but the quantity in the food may be listed elsewhere on the food package by itself or as part of a health claim.

▶ Check the Nutrition Facts for *trans* fat. If it lists 0 g, but partially hydrogenated oils, butter or other dairy fats are listed in the Ingredients list, the food may contain between 0 and 0.49g *trans* fat per serving.

TYPE OF FATTY ACID	FOOD PROPERTY	PHYSIOLOGICAL PROPERTY
All	Gives food shiny or glossy look; Contributes to texture (crispness, density, flakiness); Aids in browning; Absorbs and transports flavors; Transfers heat to food.	Component of cell membranes, brain and nervous tissue; Absorption, transportation, storage of fat soluble vitamins; Production and proper functioning of hormones that regulate blood pressure, blood clotting, immune function, smooth muscle contraction.
Saturated Fatty Acids	Solid at room temperature; Slow to oxidize; Provides texture and stability.	May increase both LDL and HDL cholesterol.
Trans Fatty Acids	Can be either man-made (partially hydrogenated oils) or naturally occurring in animal foods (meat or dairy from cows or sheep); Provides texture and stability; Slow to oxidize.	May raise total and LDL cholesterol and triglycerides.
Unsaturated Fatty Acids	Generally liquid at room temperature; More stable at high cooking temperatures.	When replacing saturated and *trans* fatty acids, may lower LDL cholesterol and improve ratio of total to HDL cholesterol; When replacing carbohydrate or saturated or *trans* fatty acids, may improve insulin sensitivity.
MUFA		
Omega-9 MUFA	Liquid at room temperature; Gets thicker/cloudy when chilled.	May help lower LDL and maintain HDL blood cholesterol levels. MUFAs may improve insulin sensitivity.
PUFA		
Omega-3 PUFA Omega-6 PUFA	Liquid at room temperature; stays liquid when refrigerated.	When replacing saturated and *trans* fatty acids, may reduce total and LDL cholesterol. Omega-6 PUFA may improve insulin sensitivity. The Omega-3 PUFA DHA assists visual and cognitive development in young infants.

Oils & Spreads

Oils are derived from plant sources, and generally provide a healthful fatty acid profile. While butter and table spreads are found in different parts of the grocery store, they can be used interchangeably with oils in some cases. Indeed, butter, shortening, and oils can also be used in processed foods, although oils are the more common choice today. The choice of oil, butter, or spread in a recipe or at the table can be based on not only health but also flavor and culinary needs.

Oils and spreads provide a surprising blend of fatty acids

▶ Olive oil is known for its high MUFA content. Canola is also a great source of MUFAs.

▶ Canola oil has the least saturated and most omega-3 fatty acids (ALA) of the common oils.

▶ Soybean oil contains a significant amount of omega-3.

▶ All cooking oils contain some saturated fatty acids.

▶ Corn, followed by soybean, oil contains the highest quantity of omega-6 fatty acids of the major cooking oils.

▶ Butter is known for its saturated fatty acids, but one-third of its fat content is unsaturated.

▶ *Trans* fatty acids have been largely eliminated from table spreads.

Storage

Protect oils from heat, light, moisture, and air, as these factors change the oil's quality over time and could accelerate spoilage. Store cooking oils in a cool, dry, dark location, such as a kitchen cabinet (but never over the refrigerator or stove). If used infrequently, store oils in the refrigerator to prolong freshness.

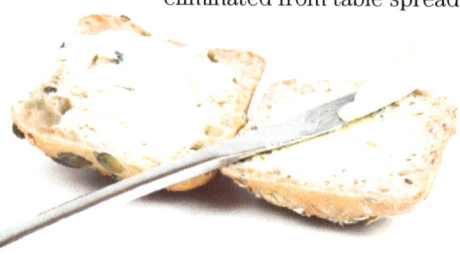

Cooking qualities

The fatty acid content of an oil, butter, or spread affects its health
and cooking qualities, and these differences matter when you are in
the kitchen. You still have a lot of flexibility based on taste preferences, though. Check out the Blending Form and Function in the
Kitchen section for details on these and other factors to consider.

An Array of Fatty Acids (g) per Serving (1tbsp) of Cooking Oils and Butter*

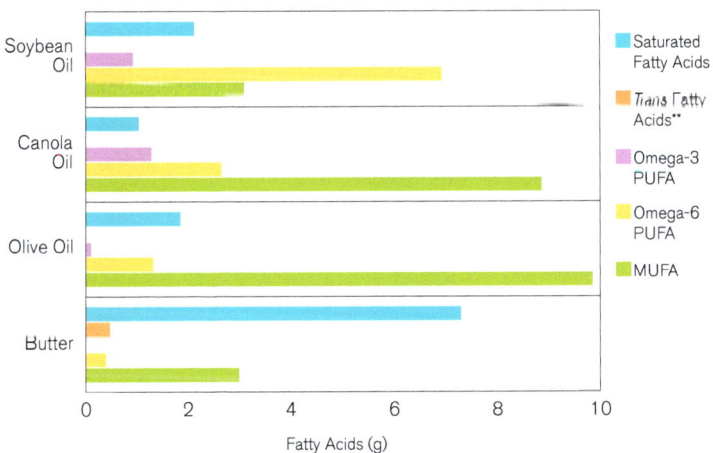

*Table spreads are not included in chart because they may contain 0-80% fat, making comparisons
difficult. Also, the fatty acid profiles of table spreads vary widely, as they include a range of combinations of liquid and in some cases solid fats.

**Trans* fatty acid content of olive oil is not reported in the USDA Food Composition Database.

What ever happened to margarine?

Did you know that federal law requires that margarine contain at least 80% fat, while the table spreads, more commonly available today, may contain 0 to 80% fat? While some contain trace amounts of partially hydrogenated oils, most table spreads contain *"0 grams of trans fatty acids per serving."* Both are made primarily from plant-derived oils.

Fun Facts about plant oils

The olive is known as the immortal tree, growing and producing fruit for hundreds of years before withering and giving life to a new tree that rises up from the old.

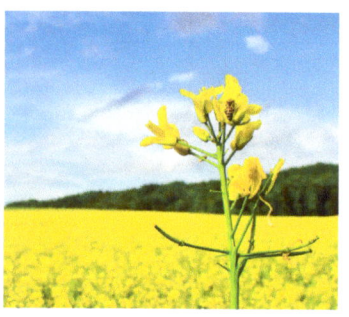

Not just for olive oil, olives can be mashed and mixed with garlic and spices to make a delectable, nutrient-rich tapenade to be enjoyed as a spread or to complement fish or chicken.

Soybeans are legumes, originating from Asia, but now grown worldwide.

Different varieties of soybeans are used for oil, whole soy foods, or soy protein food ingredients.

The canola plant is adorned with beautiful yellow flowers and small pods from which the canola seed is harvested. The tiny black seeds are crushed to produce canola oil.

Canola is in the Brassica family, along with cabbage, broccoli, and cauliflower.

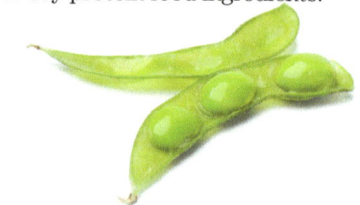

Notes

Dairy

When we think dairy, we mostly think of milk, cheese, and butter from the cow. However, hundreds of other dairy products from not only cows but also goats, as well as "milks" from plant foods (nut, soy), can be found in the dairy section of the grocery store, offering a wide variety of fatty acids and other nutrients. Eggs are another non-dairy food found in the dairy section of the supermarket. There are also countless cheeses, cultured dairy drinks and foods such as yogurt and table spreads.

Where's the "dairy" on MyPlate?

- Dairy is a separate food group on MyPlate.

- The equivalent of 3 cups of milk per day for adults is recommended. Each "cup" on MyPlate may be 1 cup of milk, yogurt, or fortified soy milk, 1 ½ oz cheese, or 2 cups cottage cheese.

- MyPlate encourages Americans to "skim the fat" by gradually switching to low-fat (1%) or fat-free milk, and to "choose cheeses with less fat," because dairy foods can be high in saturated fat.

- Cream cheese, cream, and butter are NOT part of the Dairy food group because of high levels of saturated fatty acids and little other nutritional value.

- Eggs are recommended as part of the Protein Group.

Putting ideas into action

Check out the section on Blending Form and Function in the Kitchen for ideas on choosing the right foods in the Dairy section for different cooking applications.

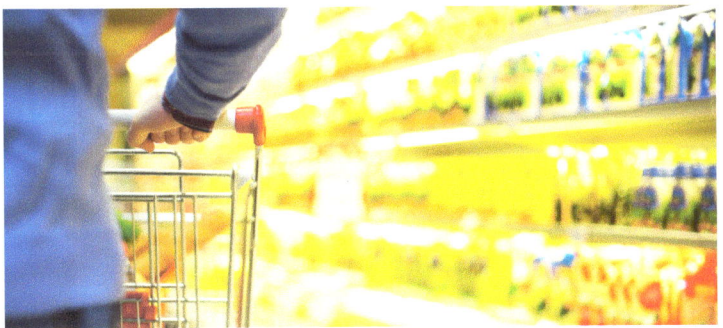

There's more to foods in the dairy section than saturated fatty acids

▶ Dairy foods include an array of fatty acids.

▶ Fat plays a role in taste and food properties, so a variety of options give you flexibility in the kitchen.

▶ Milk, yogurt, and cheese are excellent sources of calcium and protein.

▶ Low fat and fat free dairy options abound as a way to reduce intake of saturated fatty acids.

▶ Yogurts and kefir are cultured to provide probiotics, which support a healthy digestive system.

▶ Plain Greek yogurt can be higher in saturated fatty acids and protein and lower in sugar and calcium than other plain yogurts.

▶ Plant-based table spreads, as well as soy and nut alternatives to milk, yogurt, and cheese, have more unsaturated fats than dairy foods.

▶ Whole eggs have a relatively small amount of saturated fat, but limiting to one a day is recommended due to their cholesterol content. Eggs are also an excellent source of protein, choline, and certain phytochemicals.

Is coconut milk....milk?

Not if you're comparing it to cow's milk or fortified soy milk. Coconut milk is high in saturated fat and potassium, but not a good source of calcium, vitamin D, or protein. It is traditionally used in Indian food for curry and other sauces. A low fat version of coconut milk can be used to make sauces that call for butter, margarine, or shortening.

Keep it safe

▶ Avoid raw (unpasteurized) milk, dairy products, and eggs. There are no health benefits to unpasteurized milk products, and lots of risk.

▶ Refrigerate dairy products and eggs promptly when you get home from the grocery store.

▶ Remember to store mixed dishes made with dairy products or eggs in the refrigerator.

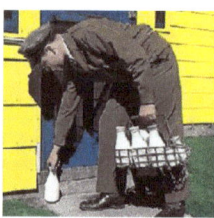

Fun facts about dairy

Home delivery of milk (The milk-man!) started in 1942 as a war conservation measure and ended in the early 60's.

The yellow color of butter comes from beta carotene, a phytochemical (the same one that makes carrots orange).

The average cow produces 6 gallons of milk a day.

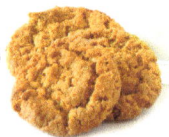

It takes more than 21 pounds of whole milk to make 1 pound of butter and 12 pounds of whole milk to make one gallon of ice cream.

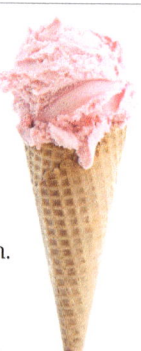

Cocoa butter, the fat in chocolate, might be expected to increase blood cholesterol levels because it contains saturated fat. However, studies have shown that consuming chocolate in moderation may not increase blood cholesterol levels.

Soy milk was patented in 1911 under the name Soja Milk, a much better term than other earlier options: "the solution of legumin," or "liquid tofu".

An Array of Fatty Acids (g) per Serving (1 c) of Yogurt

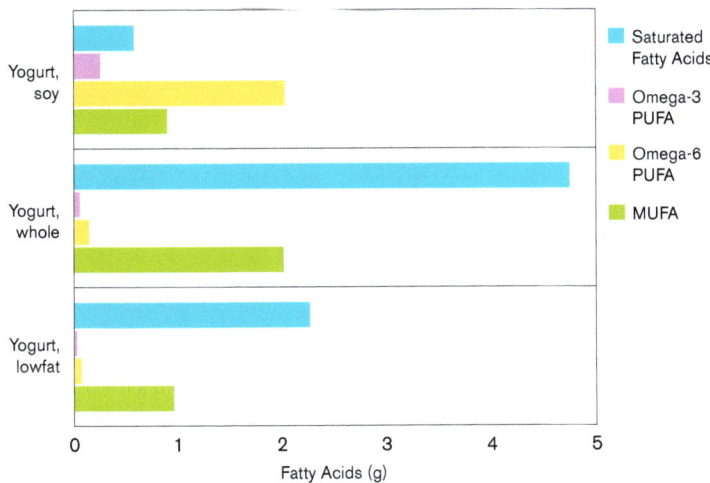

*Many dairy products contain small amounts of naturally occurring *trans* fats.

An Array of Fatty Acids (g) per Serving (1 c) of Milk

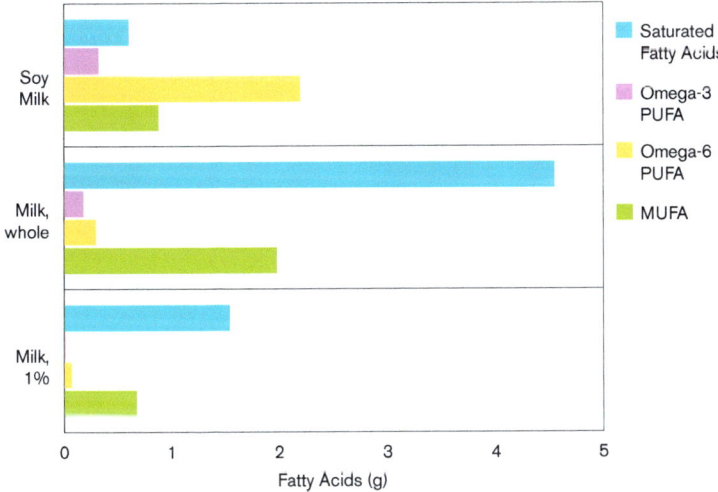

*Many dairy products contain small amounts of naturally occurring *trans* fats.

Notes

Beef, Poultry, and Pork

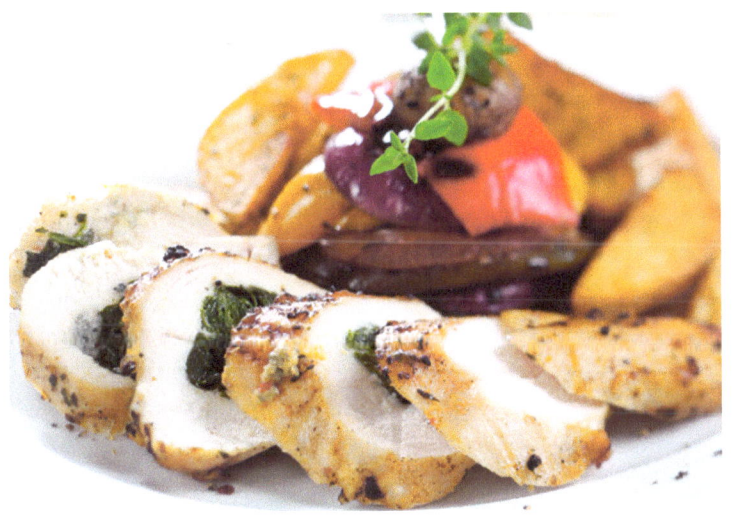

When we think of the fat in meat, we tend to think first of saturated fatty acids. However, meat, like other fat containing foods contributes an array of fatty acids to our diet. In fact, the majority of the fatty acids in most meats, including bacon, are monoun-saturated, followed by saturated.

Still, choosing lean meats (those that are lower in total fat) over those that are higher in fat is a good way to reduce our intake of saturated fatty acids. Meats with the highest total fat include 75% to 85% lean ground beef; regular sausages, hot dogs, and bacon; some luncheon meats such as regular bologna and salami; and some poultry such as duck or chicken with skin.

Safe Minimum Internal Cooking Temperatures

Meat	Temperature (°F)
Ground Beef & Pork	160
Fresh Beef	145
Poultry	165
Pork	145

Lean meats are widely available today. They have no more than 4.5 g saturated fatty acids, no more than 10 g of total fat, and less than 95 mg cholesterol. Chicken breast without skin has the least fat. There are 29 cuts of beef that meet government guidelines for lean. For pork or beef, choose cuts with the names round or loin in the name, or 95% lean ground beef (remember that 95% lean refers to the raw product, not the caloric content). And read the Nutrition Facts Label to find luncheon meats, sausage, or hot dogs that are lower in fat.

In the body

Diets that are high in saturated fats may raise LDL cholesterol, which in turn increases the risk for coronary heart disease.

Diets that are high in dietary cholesterol may also raise LDL cholesterol levels in the blood.

Fun facts about meat

The National Restaurant Association reports that the top foods eaten in restaurants are hamburgers, steaks, and roast beef.

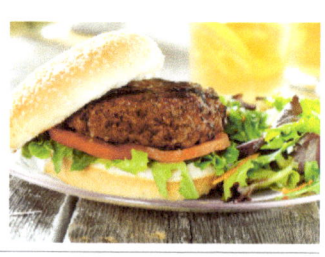

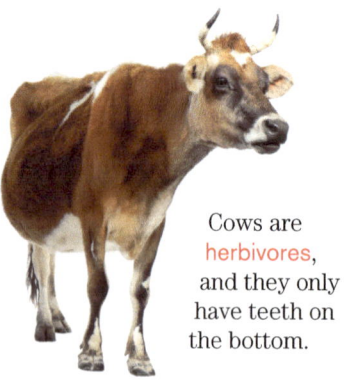

Globally, pork is the most widely consumed meat.

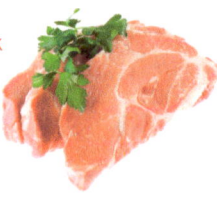

Cows are herbivores, and they only have teeth on the bottom.

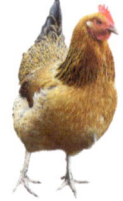

Chickens can fly only short distances, but they can run far and up to 9 miles per hour.

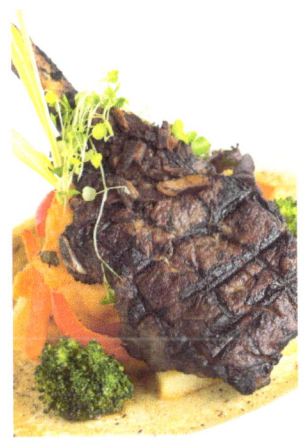

Where is meat on MyPlate?

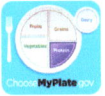

▶ The Protein food group includes meat (beef, pork, lamb), poultry, seafood, beans and peas, eggs, processed soy products, nuts, and seeds.

▶ Most adults need 5 to 7 ounces from the Protein group each day. Select a variety of protein foods to improve nutrient intake and health benefits, including 8 ounces of cooked seafood per week.

An Array of Fatty Acids (g) per Serving (3 oz) of Meats

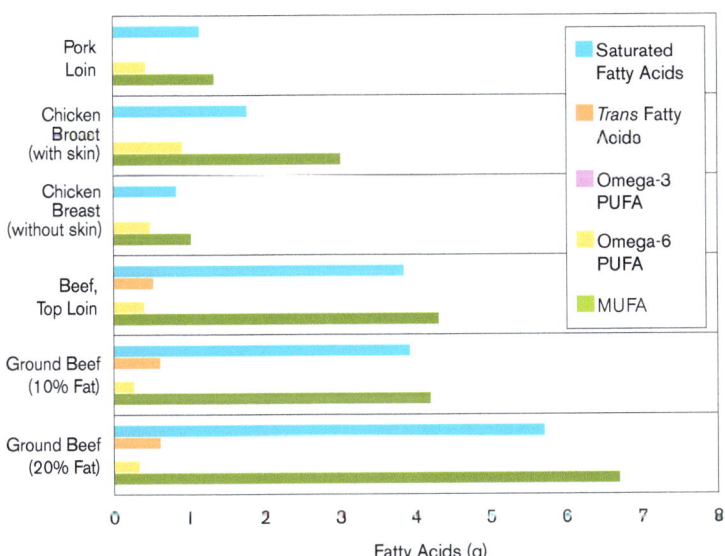

Seafood

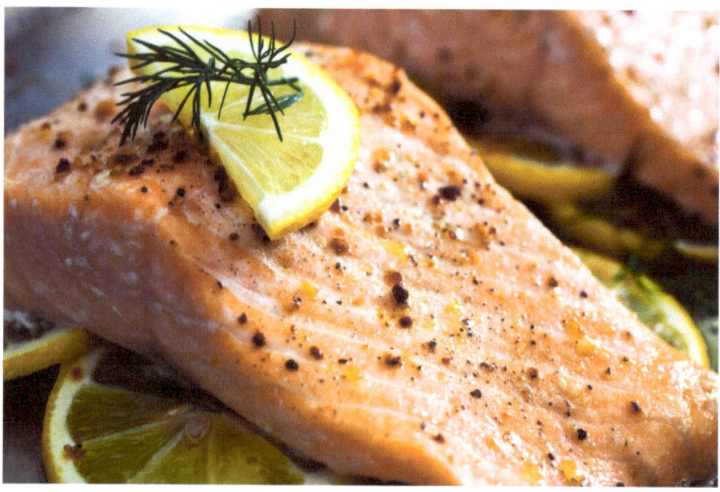

Seafood is the food perhaps most recognized for containing healthful fat. While generally low in saturated fatty acids, most seafood varieties are a good source of both MUFA and PUFA. Remember that all sources of fat contain an array of fatty acids.

Cold water oily fish contain the highest amounts of the omega-3 PUFAs EPA (eicosapentaenoic acid) and DHA (docosahexaenoic acid). Salmon, anchovies, herring, Pacific oysters, sardines, trout, and Atlantic and Pacific mackerel are the best sources of EPA and DHA.

What makes seafood such a good choice?

EPA and DHA are strongly correlated with cardiovascular disease prevention, and DHA is important for brain and vision development in infants. Plant oils and nuts provide ALA (alpha-linolenic acid), another type of omega-3 PUFA which is modestly converted to EPA and DHA in the body, and has direct health benefits as well.

Like eggs, shrimp is high in cholesterol and also a great source of protein and low in saturated fat. While the research on shrimp cholesterol and health is not definitive, it is still prudent to heed the recommendation by the Dietary Guidelines for Americans to consume 300 mg of cholesterol or less per day. A 3-oz serving of shrimp has about 170 mg cholesterol.

As for any food group or diet, variety is a key element to nutritional health. Seafood is more than shrimp and scallops. Don't forget tuna, salmon, other shellfish, tilapia, flounder, and catfish. While fresh seafood can be pricey, look for sales and areas away from the fresh seafood counter for economical options. For example, keep frozen or canned fish on hand, including salmon, tuna, and sardines, for healthful fats and high quality protein any day of the week.

Selecting and cooking

Benjamin Franklin is credited with saying, "Fish and house guests smell after 3 days." You decide on the house guests, but Ben was right about smelly fish—it should have a light sea aroma!

Cooking fish is a common source of anxiety, but it is easier than it seems. Check out the section on Blending Form and Function in the Kitchen for tips on preparation.

If you find the smell and taste of fish to be overwhelming, but you want the health benefits of those PUFAs, try a milder tasting fish. Cod, flounder, and tilapia are all great options and quick and easy to prepare. These are lower in omega-3 fatty acids, but high in protein and low in saturated fats.

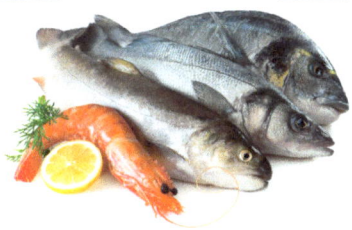

Where is seafood on MyPlate?

▶ Seafood is in the Protein group.

▶ Most adults need 5 to 7 oz from the Protein food group per day, including about 8 oz per week as fatty (omega-3-rich) fish. A 4-oz portion is a small fish filet, 8 medium sized shrimp, or 4-6 medium to large scallops.

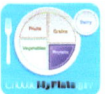

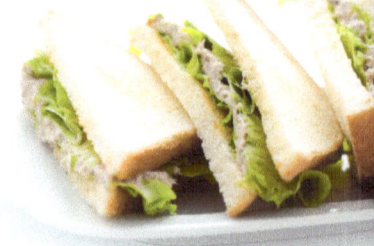

Seafood safety

▶ The health benefits of fish outweigh the potential risks of mercury contamination for most adults. Young children and pregnant women, however, should steer clear of swordfish, shark, king mackerel, and tile fish, and limit white (albacore) tuna to 6 oz per week.

▶ Seafood, depending on its source, can be at risk for environmental contaminants. For example, large fish carry mercury in their bodies which means when we consume the fish we consume the mercury as well. Contamination in local waters may also be a reality.

▶ Sushi lovers, understand that raw or partially cooked seafood poses the highest risk for foodborne illness caused by either microorganisms or naturally occurring toxins. Be sure you're getting your sushi from trusted sources.

▶ These web sites provide useful tips for selecting, handling and storing seafood.

- epa.gov/hg/advisories.htm
- water.epa.gov/learn/kids/fishkids/
- noaa.gov/deepwaterhorizon/data/seafood_safety.html (National Oceanic and Atmospheric Administration)
- foodsafety.gov
- seafoodhealthfacts.org
- State Public Health Agencies

What about fish oil supplements?

Fish oil supplements that contain EPA and DHA are an option for individuals who are looking for the health benefits, but unwilling or unable to eat fish. Food sources of nutrients are usually superior to dietary supplements due to synergy with other nutrients. ALA, the omega-3 fatty acid found in plants, can be converted to EPA and DHA in the body, but conversion rates are very low. Certain types of seaweed contain EPA and DHA, and can be included in the diet or are sometimes used to make vegan dietary supplements.

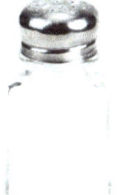

Fun facts about seafood

Despite living in salty water, most seafood (except sharks) are not high in sodium.

The oldest fish hook found dates back about 42,000 years.

Why are cold-water fish so high in unsaturated fatty acids? Fat helps to insulate the fish's body. The PUFAs are fluid even at colder temperatures, while saturated fatty acids would solidify and make it hard for fish to swim!

There are over 32,000 kinds of fish in the world today, with more species being discovered all the time.

An Array of Fatty Acids (g) per Serving (3 oz) of Seafood

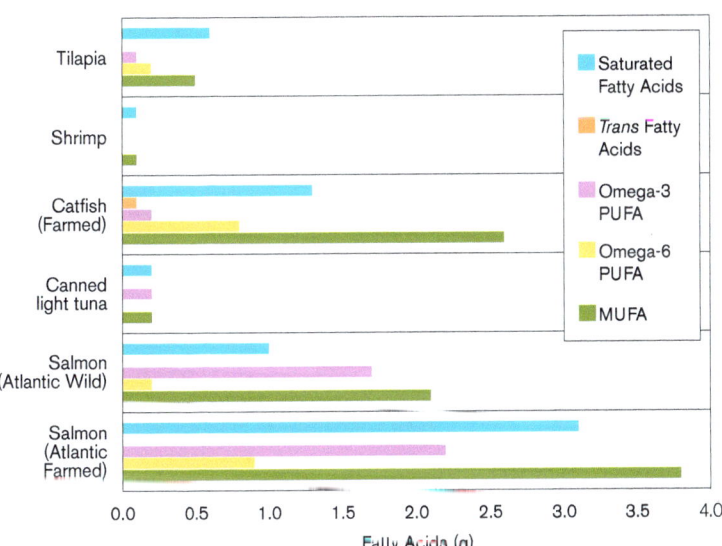

Legend:
- Saturated Fatty Acids
- *Trans* Fatty Acids
- Omega-3 PUFA
- Omega-6 PUFA
- MUFA

Categories (top to bottom): Tilapia, Shrimp, Catfish (Farmed), Canned light tuna, Salmon (Atlantic Wild), Salmon (Atlantic Farmed)

X-axis: Fatty Acids (g) — 0.0, 0.5, 1.0, 1.5, 2.0, 2.5, 3.0, 3.5, 4.0

Notes

Nuts and Seeds

Whole nuts and seeds are naturally nutrient dense foods that are portable, affordable, and easy to add to any meal or snack. Eaten whole, or ground to make nut flours or nut butters, these amazing foods have provided fiber, protein, vitamins, minerals, phytochemicals, and fats for human health and survival for thousands of years.

Most nuts and seeds contribute 70-90% of their calories as fat, with macadamia nuts, pecans, and pinenuts on the higher end, and flaxseed on the lower end. Collectively, nuts and seeds contain no cholesterol, are high in unsaturated fats (MUFA and PUFA), and are low in saturated fats. The variability is in the types of unsaturated fats. Per gram of fat, almonds and peanuts have a higher perecent of MUFAs, while walnuts and flaxseed have a higher proportion of PUFAs (omega-6 and omega-3, respectively).

All nuts are also seeds, but not all seeds are nuts.

▶ A seed is the embryonic form of a plant, that if sowed can produce a new plant. Commonly eaten seeds include sesame, sunflower, and pumpkin seeds.

▶ A nut is defined as a single seed encased in a hard shell. Common tree nuts include walnuts, almonds, cashews, macademia, filberts/hazelnuts, pistachios, and Brazil nuts.

▶ Peanuts are not nuts. They are legumes, as are pinto, black, kidney, chick peas, and other beans.

Q: Is there one best nut?

A: No, all nuts are nutrient rich and each has unique nutritional strengths. Current evidence suggests that making nuts a small but regular part of your diet can help reduce LDL cholesterol, reduce risk for developing blood clots, and improve the lining of your arteries. Collectively these benefits may add up to a decreased risk for heart disease.

Where are the nuts on MyPlate?

▶ Nuts, seeds, and legumes are all a part of the Protein Food Group on MyPlate, along with meat, poultry, seafood, eggs, peas, and soy products. 1 oz nuts or 2 tbsp nut butters are equivalent to 2 of the 5 to 7 ounces of protein foods that most people should eat each day.

▶ Nuts work well as a snack, on salads, or in main dishes.

▶ Nuts and seeds are a concentrated source of calories, so read the label for serving size to help keep calories in check.

Qualified Health Claim

▶ Scientific evidence suggests but does not prove that eating 1.5 ounces per day of most nuts (walnuts, almonds, pistachios, hazelnuts, peanuts, pecans, pine nuts) as part of a diet low in saturated fat and cholesterol may reduce the risk of heart disease.

Cooking considerations

▶ Nut and seed oils are more liquid at room temperature making them ideal for stir-frying at moderate temperatures and as additions to sauces and dressings.

▶ Nuts and nut flours can be refrigerated to extend freshness.

▶ To make your own nut flour, freeze the nuts before grinding to avoid turning the nuts into nut butter.

▶ See the section on Blending Form and Function in the Kitchen for more ideas and guidelines.

Pesto:

2-3 packed cups clean basil leaves.

¼ – ½ cup olive oil.

⅓ cup chopped nuts (pine nuts, hazelnuts, or walnuts).

½ cup grated Parmesan cheese.

2-3 cloves of fresh garlic or 1-2 tsp minced garlic.

Preparation:
Combine ¼ cup oil and all other ingredients in food processor or blender and blend until smooth. Add extra oil as needed to achieve desired consistency. Add salt and pepper as desired.

May freeze in small containers.

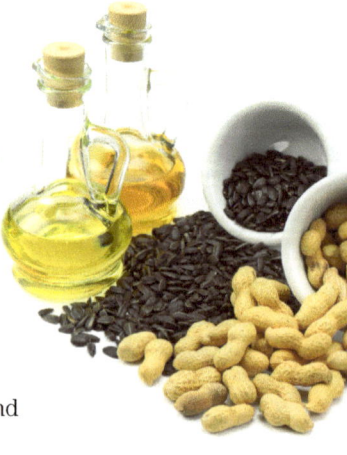

Fun facts about nuts

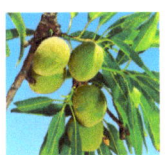

California is the almond capital with over 110,000 acres of almond trees.

The Brazil nut tree grows to a height of 150 feet and has a trunk diameter of nearly eight feet. The three to four pound pods of Brazil nuts fall to the ground when ripe, which makes gathering them a very dangerous occupation. Inside each pod, sectioned like grapefruit, are 12 to 20 seeds.

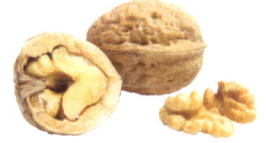

The pistachio nut cracks spontaneously when it is ripe.

Coconut, nutmeg, water chestnuts, and butternut squash are, despite their names, not nuts.

The Greeks called the walnut "the nut of Jupiter," fit for the gods.

The average walnut tree produces for 45 years.

An Array of Fatty Acids (g) per Serving (1 oz) of Nuts & Seeds

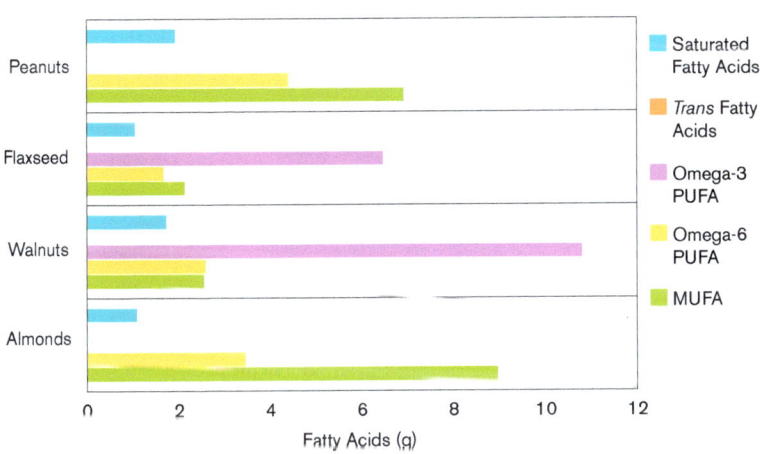

Notes

Blending Form and Function in the Kitchen

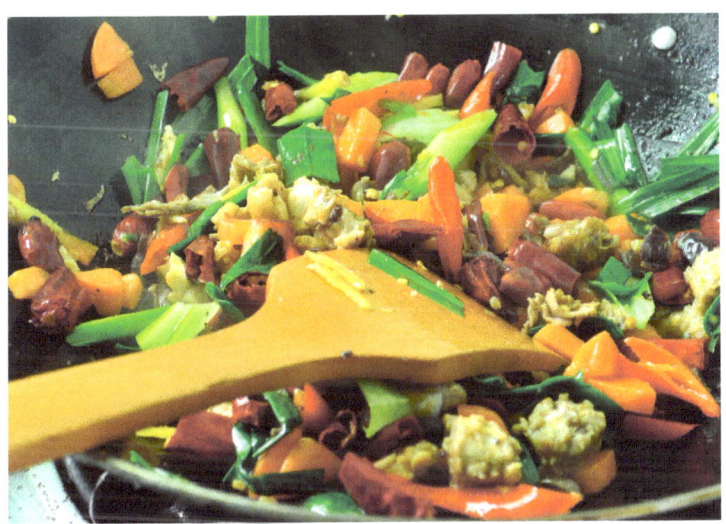

Reducing the fat level of your diet too much may drive up intake of other macronutrients, usually carbohydrates. Also, very low fat diets can reduce absorption and utilization of certain nutrients, especially essential fat-soluble vitamins A, D, E and K. Remember, dietary fat can add taste, texture and quality to food, and unsaturated fats are important for good health.

The key to a healthy intake of dietary fat is to replace saturated with unsaturated fatty acids. A source of fat that is high in MUFA and PUFA and low in saturated and *trans* fatty acids is ideal for health. Following are ways to enjoy great tasting foods while replacing saturated with unsaturated fatty acids in the kitchen

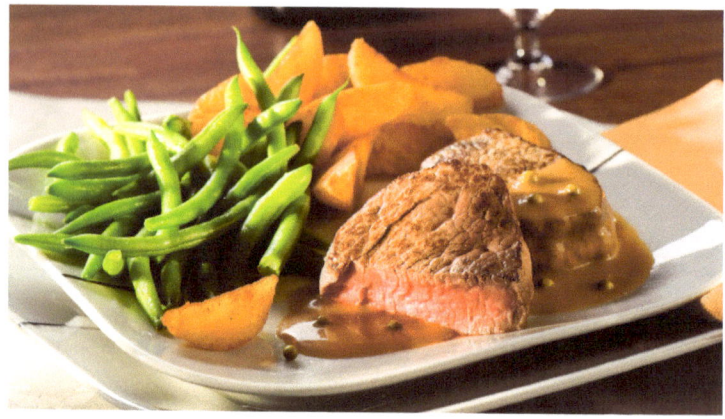

Choosing and using the right source of fat

Most cooking oils in the grocery store can be used for most cooking methods. Some, such as extra virgin olive oil, have a strong flavor that is desirable in some salad dressings or breads, but less desirable in a cake, for example. Besides flavor preferences, keep in mind the influence of smoke point (the temperature at which a fat first gives off smoke; see Table), desired food texture, length of cooking time required, and qualities of the other food ingredients.

Stir Frying, Sautéing, Frying

▶ Any liquid oil can be used in cooking at low, medium, and medium-high temperatures for shorter periods of time.

▶ Very high-heat cooking methods, such as deep frying, require fats with a higher smoke point (see Table).

▶ Butter, shortening, and margarines reach their smoke point faster than liquid oils.

▶ Table spreads are not suited for stovetop cooking because of spattering caused by the moisture content.

▶ Small pieces of vegetables or meats can be cooked quickly at a higher temperature, which reduces absorption of fat from the cooking oil, aids in browning, and reduces loss of moisture. Because of the shorter cooking time, most oils will work.

▶ If an oil or fat begins to smoke, use caution! This is a sign that the smoke is nearly hot enough to ignite. Remove from heat and let cool before properly discarding (i.e., not down the drain). Use fresh oil as needed for further cooking.

Roasting, Broiling, Grilling

▶ Cooking temperatures vary with roasting in the oven, so a range of oils can be used. A large piece of meat may be roasted at a low temperature for a long period of time, then at a high temperature at the end for browning.

▶ Broiling and grilling use very high heat in the oven or over a flame, but the cooking time is shorter. Therefore, you can choose to use a variety of oils.

▶ Vegetables may also be tossed in oil and roasted or grilled.

Baked Breads and Pastries

▶ The fat in a baking recipe can be lowered by a quarter with no substitution and minimal overall impact on quality and taste. Using less butter in a cookie recipe, for example, would decrease spreading.

▶ Liquid oil can replace butter or shortening in equal amounts. However, some baked goods that are very flaky, such as a croissant or biscuit, may require solid fats, such as butter or shortening. (Remember: these products may contain *trans* and/or saturated fatty acids)

▶ Plain yogurt, applesauce, or egg whites may be substituted for fat in a baking recipe. Expect some changes in taste and texture, so test out small modifications.

▶ Nut flour (especially almond flour) can be used as a substitute for ¼ of the wheat flour used in cookies and baked foods.

▶ Due to the different types of fats in nut flours, their use in cooking and baking may vary.

▶ To make your own nut flour, freeze the nuts first to prevent turning the nuts into nut butter, then grind with coffee grinder.

Salad Dressings & Toppings

▶ Choose salad dressings made with liquid vegetable oils over creamy full-fat varieties.

▶ Make your own salad dressing with canola, olive, or soybean oils, combined with your preferred vinegar, herbs and spices, using taste as your guide. Canola or soybean oils would work well in a fruit vinaigrette, while extra virgin olive would be more suited to an herb vinaigrette.

▶ Canola, and soybean oils can be refrigerated for extended freshness without solidifying. Oils may become cloudy when refrigerated, but this is harmless and will clear when the product is warmed to room temperature.

▶ Nut or seed oils can also be used, especially if a unique flavor from the oil is desired.

▶ Top your salad with chopped nuts.

▶ If you add cheese to your salad, use small amounts of feta, blue, gorgonzola, or goat cheeses.

Sandwiches

▶ Choose lower fat cheeses, or thinly sliced portions. Try new flavors with Swiss, provolone, or gouda.

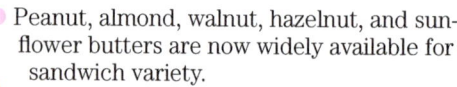

▶ Peanut, almond, walnut, hazelnut, and sunflower butters are now widely available for sandwich variety.

▶ Pesto makes a unique sandwich spread, adding healthful fats and protein to a roasted vegetable sandwich.

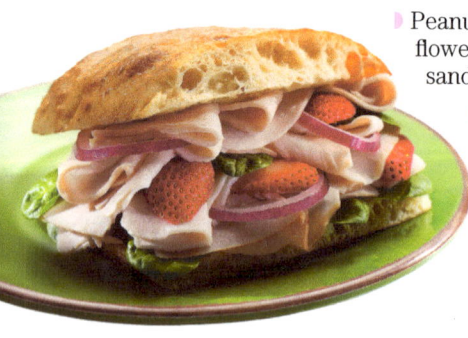

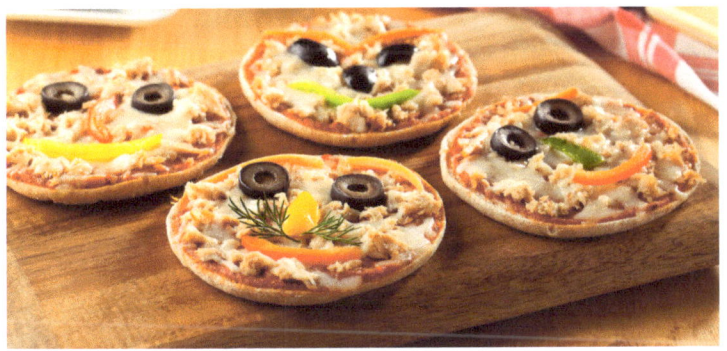

Cheesy Choices

▶ Choose lower-fat versions of cheddar and mozzarella when using in mixed food recipes.

▶ When full fat cheeses are preferred, use less without sacrificing flavor:

- select stronger favored cheeses such as sharp/aged cheddar, blue, asiago;

- grate or shred cheese to spread it more evenly than solid chucks or slices;

- reduce the amount of cheese in a casserole, while sprinkling a bit on top for "visible" flavor in each bite.

Seafood

▶ Remember, fresh fish should have a light sea air smell, and should be cooked within a day or two of purchase.

▶ If you want to buy fish in advance choose frozen or canned fish.

▶ Cooking fish is a common source of anxiety, but is actually relatively quick and easy. The best approach is to start with a recipe and use your meat thermometer to ensure doneness without overcooking.

Meats

▶ Ground nuts can be used as meat breading or mixed into your favorite lean meat or veggie burger recipes.

▶ Broil or sauté instead of frying in a lot of oil.

▶ Use a roasting pan with a drain rack to allow fats to drip off during cooking process.

▶ Remove the skin and trim the fat before roasting. Or, remove skin and trim fat following roasting in order to preserve some of the flavor and cooking qualities of fat.

Dips and Toppings

▶ Chopped nuts are great additions to yogurt, oatmeal, salads, baked goods, and vegetable and stir fry dishes.

▶ Try nut butters for fruit and vegetable dips.

▶ Choose low fat sour cream, yogurt, or cottage cheese to make dips with lots of spices, herbs, or fruits for flavor.

Storage and Freshness

Unsaturated fats are more prone to oxidation and spoilage than saturated fats, although a few tips will keep your healthful fats fresh:

▶ Most plant oils can be refrigerated to extend freshness.

▶ Oils with a high omega-3 PUFA content, such as walnut and flaxseed, should always be refrigerated.

▶ Oils with high saturated fatty acid or MUFA content may become cloudy when refrigerated, but return to a clear liquid when at room temperature.

▶ Nut flours must be refrigerated, and nuts will remain fresh longer if refrigerated.

▶ Remember that dairy, eggs, meats, and seafood are perishable, so pay attention to expiration dates and follow the "Clean, Separate, Cook, Chill" rules to keep foods safe. See foodsafety.gov for more food safety information!

Cooking Uses and Smoke Points of Various Cooking Oils and Solid Fats

Fats or Oils	Suggested Cooking Uses	Primary Fatty Acids	Smoke Point °F
Butter	Baking, browning	Saturated	300°F
Canola Oil	Stir-frying, baking, salad dressings, marinades. Substitute for melted butter, margarine or shortening. Mild flavor	MUFA	468°F
Corn Oil	Frying. Mild flavor.	PUFA	455°F
Lard	Baking and frying	Saturated	464°F
Olive Oil, Refined and/or Virgin*	Pan frying, searing, stir-frying, sautéing, grilling, broiling, baking, dipping	MUFA	410°F
Olive Oil, Extra Virgin*	Salad dressings, quick sauté.	MUFA	320 to 375°F
Rice Bran Oil	Frying, sautéing, salad dressings, baking, dipping oils	MUFA	444°F
Safflower Oil, Traditional	Margarine, mayonnaise, salad dressings	PUFA	510°F
Shortening, Vegetable	Baking	Saturated or *trans*	325°F
Soybean Oil (Often sold as "Vegetable Oil")	Margarine, salad dressings, shortening	PUFA	464°F
Mid Oleic Sunflower Oil	Cooking, margarine, salad dressings, shortening	PUFA	412°F

*Due to the wide range of olive oils available, smoke points may vary widely.

Sources: http://iseo.org/httpdocs/Publications/Smoke-Fire_Chart_0310.pdf; http://www.canolainfo.org/news/latest_news.php?detail=726;

The Culinary Institute of America (1996) at http://drinc.ucdavis.edu/dairychem7_new.htm; http://www.internationaloliveoil.org/web/aa-ingles/oliveWorld/aceite3.html

Notes